AIR FRYER QUICK START GUIDE

A Straightforward Guide to Quick, Easy and Tasty Air Fryer Recipes for Everyday Cooking

Hollie McCarthy RDN

deemed liable for any hardship or damages that may befall them after undertaking information described herein.

Additionally, the information in the following pages is intended only for informational purposes and should thus be thought of as universal. As befitting its nature, it is presented without assurance regarding its prolonged validity or interim quality. Trademarks that are mentioned are done without written consent and can in no way be considered an endorsement from the trademark holder.

Table of Content

Introduction

Welcome to the air fryer guide!

The air fryer is one of the most impressive and useful inventions of the decade. With this machine, you can reduce the amount of grease you consume from traditional dishes and snacks such as chicken nuggets and French fries. Goes without saying that cooking time is considerably reduced!

It is a multi-cooker that performs more than functions. The air fryer enables you to cook a wide variety of dishes including meat, fish, eggs, grain, poultry, beans, cakes, yogurt and vegetables etc. What Serves: it exceptional is because you can use different cooking programs such as a steamer, rice cooker, sauté pan, and even a warming pot, thus saving more time, money, and space than buying any other kitchen appliances.

The Air fryer Serves: as a multi-use programmable appliance can help create easy, fast and flavorful recipes with the ability to apply different cooking settings all in one pot. It was developed by Canadian technology experts seeking to be the ultimate kitchen mate, from stir-frying, pressure cooking, slow cooking and yogurt and cake making. It was created to serve as a one-stop shop to allow home cooks prepare a tasty meal with the press of a button. You can cook almost everything in this fryer.

The air fryer uses an ingenious combination of both Directions, differing from the convection oven because heat circulates everywhere (vice rising to the top) through the fan, and not through the turbo because there is typically no heating element in the top of a fryer from where the heat comes out. They use electrical energy to create their heat; a lot of power!

Many people still have their doubts regarding the importance of this machine, and what a healthy alternative it can be. Despite its popularity, in some regions it has not yet reached the peak of its use. It is very likely that in a short time new brands will emerge in other regions and the air fryer will grow in popularity across the nation.

The use of this tool consists of cooking something without boiling the product in oil or fat. At most, the maximum oil needed by the air fryer is a tablespoon, which is used to prevent the food from sticking and forming an overdone crust.

What is an air fryer?

An air fryer works with "fast air technology." This means that there is a highspeed circulation of hot air that cocoons the food you cook.

During this process, the air fryer prepares the food evenly, all the while giving it a "fried" taste and texture without ever actually having to fry anything in grease.

While many people and regions near and far are familiar with this tool, the electric fryer is even crossing the waters. They are even found commonly in Europe and Australia!

The air fryer is similar in concept to a convection oven or a turbo grill, although the fryer still differs slightly from both appliances. Convection ovens and turbo broilers depend on different heating Directions and are often larger and bulkier appliances to use when cooking your food.

In this book, we will explore the variety of easy delicious dishes you can cook with your air fryer. We will explore a wide variety of dishes, from breakfast to dinner, soups to stews, desserts to appetizers, meat to beef, side dishes to vegetables and use a healthy ingredient in the process. The vast majority of the recipes can be prepared and served in less than 45 minutes. Each recipe is written with the exact cooking Directions and ingredients required to prepare dishes that will satisfy and nourish you. Once you try the delish dishes in this cookbook, you and your air fryer are sure to become inseparable too.

It's important to think outside the box when it comes to trying out recipes in your air fryer. From roasted vegetables to empanadas, to baked eggs and vegan brownies, there's an option for everyone when you use your air fryer.

This cookbook is for people who want to create tasty dishes without spending all day in the kitchen. Most of the recipes can be prepared in 15 minutes or less. And most of them can be on the table in under an hour. With today's busy lifestyles, I know this is important to most of you.

In keeping with the latest health trends and diets, the recipes also include complete nutrition information. As a plus, there are recipes for those on a Vegan Diet as well as Mediterranean diet.

Let's delve in!

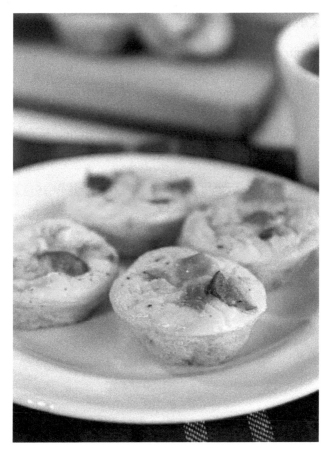

Serves: 4

INGREDIENTS

- 4 crusty rolls
- 5 eggs, beaten
- A pinch of salt
- ½ tsp thyme, dried
- 3 strips precooked bacon, chopped

- 2 tbsp heavy cream
- 4 Gouda cheese mini wedges, thin slices

DIRECTIONS

1. Preheat your air fryer 330 degrees F. Cut the tops off the rolls and remove the inside with your fingers. Line the rolls with a slice of cheese and press down, so the cheese conforms to the inside of the roll. In a bowl, mix eggs with heavy cream, bacon, thyme, salt, and pepper.

2. Stuff the rolls with the egg mixture. Lay the rolls in your air fryer's cooking basket and bake for 8 to 12 minutes or until the eggs become puffy and the roll shows a golden brown texture.

Per serving: Calories: 499; Carbs:46g; Fat: 24g; Protein: 26g

Air Fried Calzone

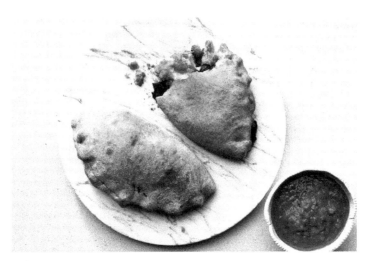

Serves: 4

INGREDIENTS

- Pizza dough
- 4 oz cheddar cheese, grated
- 1 oz mozzarella cheese
- 1 oz bacon, diced
- 2 cups cooked and shredded turkey
- 1 egg, beaten
- 1 tsp thyme
- 4 tbsp tomato paste
- 1 tsp basil
- 1 tsp oregano
- Salt and pepper, to taste

DIRECTIONS

1. Preheat the air fryer to 350 degrees F. Divide the pizza dough into 4 equal pieces so you have the dough for 4 small pizza crusts. Combine the tomato paste, basil, oregano, and thyme, in a small bowl.

2. Brush the mixture onto the crusts just make sure not to go all the way and avoid brushing near the edges on one half of each crust, place ½ turkey, and season the meat with some salt and pepper.

3. Top the meat with some bacon. Combine the cheddar and mozzarella and divide it between the pizzas, making sure that you layer only one half of the dough.

4. Brush the edges of the crust with the beaten egg. Fold the crust and seal with a fork. Cook for 10 minutes.

Per serving: Calories: 339; Carbs:10.6 g; Fat: 17.3 g; Protein: 33.6 g

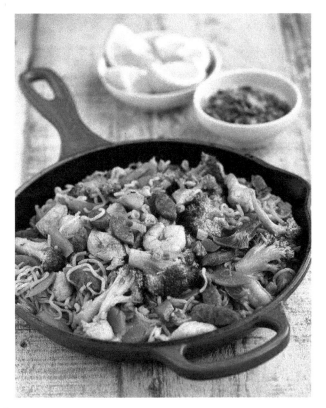

Serves: 4

INGREDIENTS

- 4 boneless and skinless chicken breasts cut into cubes
- 2 carrots, sliced
- 1 red bell pepper, cut into strips
- 1 yellow bell pepper, cut into strips
- 1 cup snow peas
- 15 oz broccoli florets
- 1 scallion, sliced

SAUCE:

- 3 tbsp soy sauce
- 2 tbsp oyster sauce
- 1 tbsp brown sugar
- 1 tsp sesame oil
- 1 tsp cornstarch
- 1 tsp sriracha
- 2 garlic cloves, minced
- 1 tbsp grated ginger
- 1 tbsp rice wine vinegar

DIRECTIONS

1. Preheat the air fryer to 370 degrees F. Place the chicken, bell peppers, and carrot, in a bowl. In another bowl, combine the sauce ingredients. Coat the chicken mixture with the sauce.

2. Place on a lined baking sheet and cook for 5 minutes. Add snow peas and broccoli and cook for an additional 8 to 10 minutes. Serve garnished with scallion.

Per serving: Calories: 277; Carbs:15.6 g; Fat: 4.4 g; Protein: 43.1 g

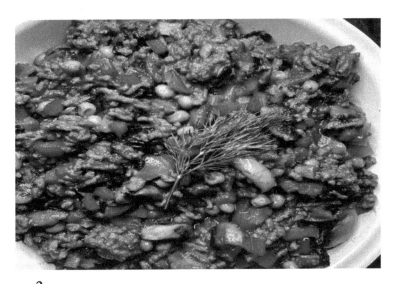

Serves: 2

Ingredients

- ½ lb ground lamb meat

- ½ cup onion, chopped

- ½ tablespoon garlic

- ½ tablespoon minced ginger

- ¼ teaspoon turmeric

- ¼ teaspoon ground coriander

- ½ teaspoon salt

- ¼ teaspoon cumin

- ¼ teaspoon cayenne pepper

Directions

1. Set the Air Fryer to 'sauté' mode.

2. Add the onions, garlic, and ginger, and sauté for 5 minutes.

3. Add the remaining ingredients to the pot and secure the lid.

4. Cook on the 'manual' function for 15 minutes at high pressure.

5. After the beep, 'natural release' the steam for 15 minutes.

6. Remove the lid and serve immediately.

Nutrition Values (Per Serving): Calories: 343 | Carbohydrate: 4.8g |
Protein: 28.7g | Fat: 22.5g

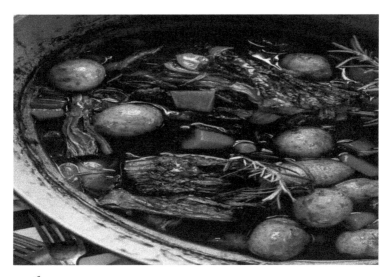

Serves: 6

Ingredients

- 2½ lbs. beef roast

- 1 teaspoon garlic powder

- 1 teaspoon onion powder

- 2 tablespoons olive oil

- 1 teaspoon salt

- ½ teaspoon black pepper

- 2 tablespoons Worcestershire sauce

- 3 cups beef broth

- 2 lbs. potatoes, quartered

- ½ lb. carrots, peeled and cut into chunks

Directions

1. Turn on the Air Fryer and set it to 'sauté.' In a bowl, mix the salt, pepper, garlic powder, and onion powder.

2. Rub the mixture all over the roast to coat all sides using your hands.

3. Drizzle oil in the pot and when the oil is heated, place the roast and sear for 4-5 minutes on each side.

4. Switch the Air Fryer to 'pressure cook' on high and set to 55-65 minutes depending on how large your pieces are (65 minutes to be safe)

5. Add the potatoes, carrots and pour the beef broth and Worcestershire sauce over everything.

6. Lock the lid of the Air Fryer making sure the vent is set to the sealed position.

7. Once done, 'Natural release' the steam for 10 minutes, then remove the lid.

8. Shred or chunk the roast. Garnish with fresh parsley if desired and serve warm with the veggies.

Nutrition Values (Per Serving): Calories: 456| Carbohydrate: 17g| Protein: 57.5g| Fat: 12.1g

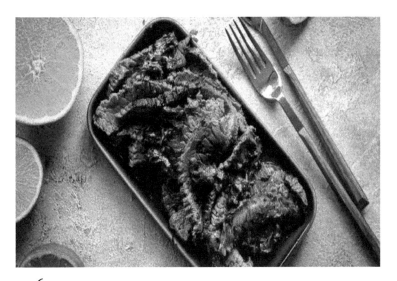

Serves: 6

Ingredients

- 2 lbs beef stew meat

- ¾ tablespoon chili powder

- 2 tablespoon salt

- 1½ tablespoons olive oil

- ½ cup beef bone broth

- ½ large onion, sliced

- ¾ tablespoon cumin

- 1 tablespoon lemon juice

- 1½ oz. tomato paste

Directions

1. Season the stew meat with salt, cumin, and chili powder.

2. Select the 'sauté' function on your Air Fryer to heat the oil.

3. Place the beef in the pot and secure the lid.

4. Cook on 'manual' function for 35 minutes at high pressure.

5. Once done 'Natural release' the steam and remove the lid.

6. Add the remaining ingredients and let it sit for 5 minutes.

7. Serve warm.

Nutrition Values (Per Serving): Calories: 408| Carbohydrate: 13.4g| Protein: 58.6g| Fat: 15.3g

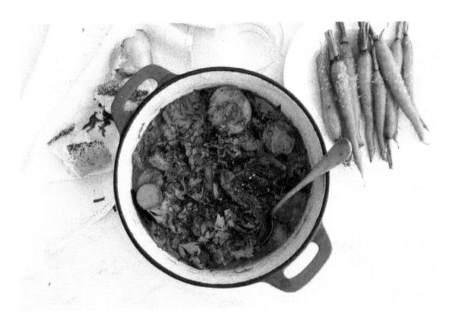

Serves: 8

Ingredients

- 8 lamb shoulder chops, cubed

- 4 cups water

- 4 tablespoons olive oil

- 8 large onions, sliced into thin rounds

- 9 large carrots, chunked

- 4 sprigs thyme

- 2 teaspoons salt

- 2 teaspoons black pepper

Directions

1. Select the 'sauté' on the Air Fryer and heat the oil in it.

2. Add the lamb chops and cook until they turn brown.

3. Transfer the chops to a plate.

4. Pour the water into the pot and add the thyme.

5. Put the chops back into the pot and arrange the vegetable over them.

6. Sprinkle with some salt and pepper and secure the lid.

7. Cook for 15 minutes on 'manual' at high pressure.

8. After the beep 'Natural release' the steam, then remove the lid.

9. Serve warm.

Nutrition Values (Per Serving): Calories: 325 | Carbohydrate: 22.5g | Protein: 24.4g | Fat: 16.2g

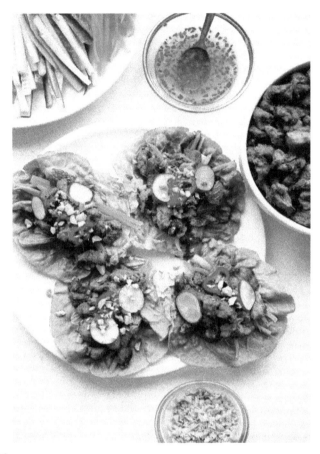

Serves: 6

Ingredients

- 3 lbs bone-in pork shoulder
- ¾ teaspoon ground cumin
- 1¼ pinches cayenne
- ½ teaspoon black pepper
- ½ teaspoon dried oregano

- ¾ teaspoon garlic powder

- ¾ teaspoon sea salt

- 1¼ tablespoon olive oil

- 1¼ onions, chopped

- 1¼ oranges, juiced

- 2 cups water

- 6 lettuce leaves

Directions

1. Put all the ingredients in except the lettuce with the pork and mix them well. Refrigerate overnight.

2. Heat the oil in the Air Fryer using the 'sauté' function.

3. Put the marinated pork into the oil and sear for 10 minutes.

4. Pour in 2 cups of water and secure the lid.

5. Select the 'manual' function and cook for 45 minutes at medium pressure.

6. Release the pressure for 10 minutes using 'Natural release'.

7. Serve the cooked pork on lettuce leaves.

Nutrition Values (Per Serving): Calories: 514| Carbohydrate: 7.6g| Protein: 39.2g| Fat: 35.5g

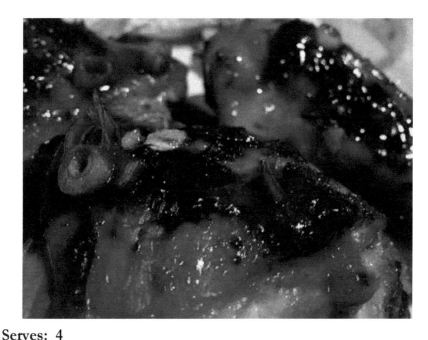

Serves: 4

Ingredients:

- 4 chicken breasts
- 4 passion fruits; halved, deseeded and pulp reserved
- 1 tbsp. whiskey
- 2-star anise
- 2 oz. maple syrup
- 1 bunch chives; chopped • Salt and black pepper to the taste

Directions:

1. Heat a pan with the passion fruit pulp over medium heat, add whiskey, star anise, maple syrup, and chives; stir well, simmer for 5-6 minutes and take off the heat.

2. Season chicken with salt and pepper put in the preheated air fryer and cook at 360 °F, for 10 minutes; flipping halfway. Divide chicken on plates heat the sauce a bit, drizzle it over chicken and serve.

Nutrition Facts (Per Serving): Calories: 374; Fat: 8; Fiber: 22; Carbs: 34; Protein: 37

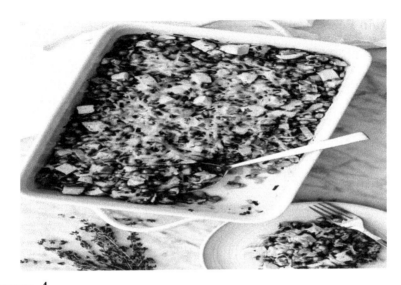

Serves: 4

Ingredients:

- 2 lbs. turkey breasts; skinless, boneless • 1 yellow onion; chopped

- 1 celery stalk; chopped.

- 1/2 cup peas

- 1 cup chicken stock

- 1 cup cream of mushrooms soup

- 1 cup bread cubes

- Salt and black pepper to the taste

Directions:

1. In a pan that fits your air fryer, mix turkey with salt, pepper, onion, celery, peas, and stock, introduce in your air fryer and cook at 360 °F, for 15 minutes.

2. Add bread cubes and cream of mushroom soup; stir toss and cook at 360 °F, for 5 minutes more. Divide among plates and serve hot.

Nutrition Facts (Per Serving): Calories: 271; Fat: 9; Fiber: 9; Carbs: 16; Protein: 7

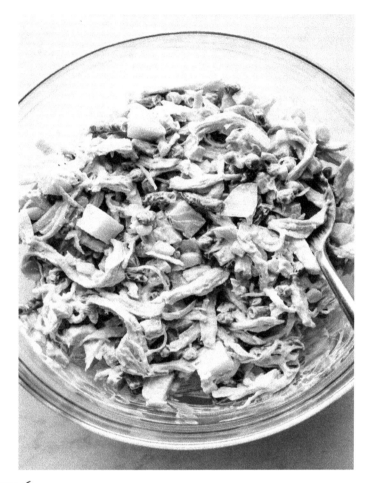

Serves: 6

Ingredients:

- 29 oz. chicken stock

- 2 cups whipping cream

- 40 oz. chicken pieces; boneless and skinless

- 3 tbsp. butter; melted

- 1/2 cup yellow onion; chopped.

- 3/4 cup red peppers; chopped

- 1 bay leaf

- 8 oz. mushrooms; chopped

- 17 oz. asparagus; trimmed

- 3 tsp. thyme; chopped.

- Salt and black pepper to the taste

Directions:

1. Heat a pan with the butter over medium heat, add onion and peppers; stir and cook for 3 minutes.

2. Add stock, bay leaf, salt, and pepper bring to a boil, and simmer for 10 minutes.

3. Add asparagus, mushrooms, chicken, cream, thyme, salt, and pepper to the taste; stir, introduce in your air fryer, and cook at 360 °F, for 15 minutes. Divide chicken and veggie mix between plates and serve.

Nutrition Facts (Per Serving): Calories: 360; Fat: 27; Fiber: 13; Carbs: 24; Protein: 47

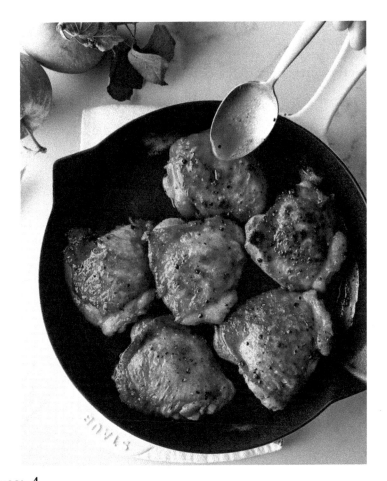

Serves: 4

Ingredients:

- 6 chicken thighs; bone-in and skin on

- 1 sweet potato; cubed

- 2 apples; cored and sliced • 1 tbsp. olive oil

- 1 tbsp. rosemary; chopped.

- 2/3 cup apple cider

- 1 tbsp. mustard

- 2 tbsp. honey

- 1 tbsp. butter

- Salt and black pepper to the taste

Directions:

1. Heat a pan that fits your air fryer with half of the oil over medium-high heat, add cider, honey, butter, and mustard, whisk well, bring to a simmer, take off heat, add chicken and toss well.

2. In a bowl, mix potato cubes with rosemary, apples, salt, pepper, and the rest of the oil; toss well and add to the chicken mix.

3. Place pan in your air fryer and cook at 390 °F, for 14 minutes. Divide everything between plates and serve.

Nutrition Facts (Per Serving): Calories: 241; Fat: 7; Fiber: 12; Carbs:28; Protein: 22

Duck Breasts with Orange Sauce

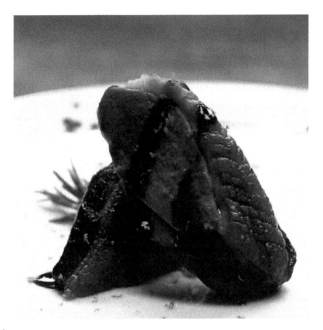

Serves: 4

Ingredients:

- 2 duck breasts; skin on and halved

- 2 cups chicken stock

- 2 cups orange juice

- 2 tsp. pumpkin pie spice

- 2 tbsp. olive oil

- 2 tbsp. butter

- 1/2 cup honey

- 2 tbsp. sherry vinegar

- 4 cups red wine

- Salt and black pepper to the taste

Directions:

1. Heat a pan with the orange juice over medium heat, add honey; stir well and cook for 10 minutes.

2. Add wine, vinegar, stock, pie spice, and butter; stir well, cook for 10 minutes more and take off the heat.

3. Season duck breasts with salt and pepper, rub with olive oil, place in the preheated air fryer at 370 °F, and cook for 7 minutes on each side. 4. Divide duck breasts on plates, drizzle wine and orange juice all over, and serve right away.

Nutrition Facts (Per Serving): Calories: 300; Fat: 8; Fiber: 12; Carbs:24; Protein: 11

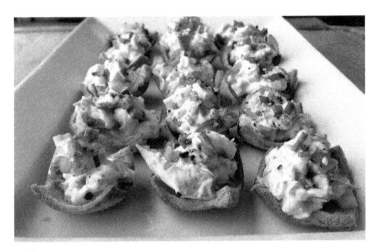

Serves: 4

Ingredients:

- 2 lobster tails, shells removed

- 2 tbsp butter

- Salt and pepper to taste

- 4 tbsp mayo

- 1 tbsp lemon juice

- 4 big salad leaves

- 4 hot dog buns

Directions:

1. Preheat your cooking machine to 135 degrees F.

2. Sprinkle the lobster tails with salt and pepper.

3. Put the tails into the vacuum bag and add the butter.

4. Seal the bag and set the timer for 1 hour.

5. When the time is up, carefully remove the cooked lobster tails, let them cool down a bit and chop them into bitesize pieces.

6. Mix the lobster pieces with mayo, sprinkle with lemon juice.

7. Put 1 big salad leave into each hot dog bun, lay the lobster mayo mixture on each leave, and serve.

Nutrition per serving: Calories: 260, Protein: 21 g, Fats: 16 g, Carbs: 8 g

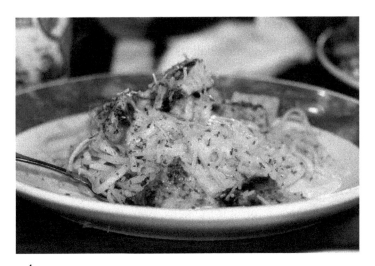

Serves: 4

Ingredients:

- 2 lobster tails, shell removed

- 1 shallot, minced

- 1 tbsp unsalted butter, melted

- 1 tbsp Cajun seasoning

- 2 garlic cloves, minced

- 4 tbsp lemon juice

- 1 tbsp lemon zest

- Salt and pepper to taste

- 2 cups dry white wine

- 4 tbsp freshly chopped parsley

- Cooked spaghetti (for 4 persons)

Directions:

1. Preheat your cooking machine to 135 degrees F.

2. Season the lobster tails with Cajun, salt, and pepper, and put them into the vacuum bag. Add shallots and butter.

3. Seal the bag, put it into the water bath, and set the timer for 1 hour.

4. Carefully chop the cooked lobster tails into bite-size pieces and pour them together with all cooking liquid into a medium pot.

5. Add the lemon juice, lemon zest and 2 cups dry white wine to the pot.

6. Simmer the mixture until it thickens, pour the sauce over the cooked penne and serve with chopped fresh parsley.

Nutrition per serving: Calories: 450, Protein: 19 g, Fats: 17 g, Carbs: 55 g

Aromatic Shrimps

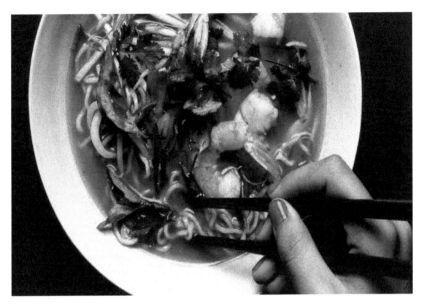

Serves: 2

Ingredients:

- 1 pound large shrimps, peeled and deveined
- 1 tsp olive oil
- Any aromatics of your choice
- Salt to taste
- 1 tbsp lemon juice (optional)

Directions:

1. Preheat your cooking machine to 125 degrees F.
2. Season the shrimps with salt and put them into the vacuum bag.
3. Add 1 tsp olive oil and aromatics.
4. Seal the bag, put it into the water bath, and set the timer for 30 minutes.

5. Serve with any sauce of your choice or sprinkled with lemon juice.

Nutrition per serving: Calories: 202, Protein: 27 g, Fats: 1 g, Carbs: 9 g

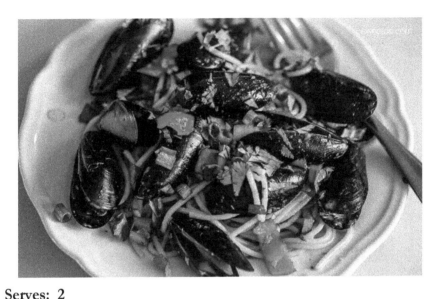

Serves: 2

Ingredients:

- 2 pounds mussels in their shells

- 1 cup dry white wine

- 2 garlic cloves, chopped

- 4 tbsp butter Salt to taste

Directions:

1. Preheat your cooking machine to 194 degrees F.

2. Season the mussels with salt and put them into the vacuum bag.

3. Reduce the air in the bag to 30% (70% of vacuum) otherwise the shell won't open.

4. Add dry white wine, garlic cloves, and butter

5. Seal the bag, put it into the water bath, and set the timer for 15 minutes.

6. Serve sprinkled with lemon juice.

Nutrition per serving: Calories: 370, Protein: 18 g, Fats: 25 g, Carbs: 18 g

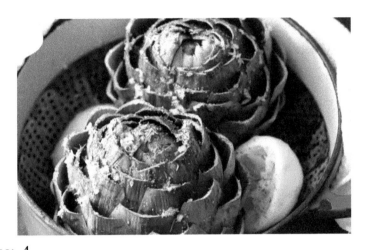

Serves: 4

Ingredients

- 4 artichokes, trimmed

- 2 lemons, one juiced, and one sliced

- ½ tablespoon peppercorns, whole

- 1 ½ garlic cloves, chopped

- ½ tablespoons olive oil

- 2 cups water

- Salt and pepper to taste

Directions

1. Pour the water and peppercorns into the insert of the Air Fryer.

2. Place the steamer trivet inside.

3. Arrange the artichokes over the trivet.

4. Secure the lid and select the "Manual" function with low pressure for 5 minutes.

5. After the beep, do a Natural release and remove the lid.

6. Strain the artichokes and return them to the pot.

7. Add the oil and all the remaining ingredients back into the Instant Pot, and then "Sauté" for 5 minutes while stirring.

8. Serve hot.

Nutrition Values (Per Serving): Calories: 103, Carbohydrate: 20.5g, Protein: 5.7g, Fat: 2.1g

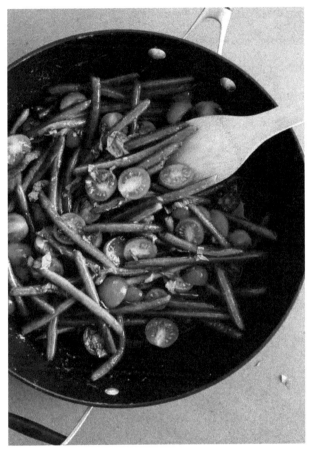

Serves: 8

Ingredients

- 2 tablespoons olive oil

- 2 garlic cloves, crushed

- 4 cups fresh tomatoes, diced

- 2 lbs. green beans

- Salt to taste

Directions

1. Add the oil and garlic to the Air Fryer and "Sauté" for 1 minute.

2. Stir in tomatoes and sauté for another 1 minute.

3. Set the steamer trivet in the pot and arrange green beans over it.

4. Secure the lid and select the "Manual" function with high pressure for 5 minutes.

5. After it is done, do a Natural release to release the steam.

6. Remove the lid and the trivet along with green beans.

7. Add the beans to the tomatoes in the pot.

8. Sprinkle salt and stir well. Serve hot.

Nutrition Values (Per Serving): Calories: 82, Carbohydrate: 11.8g, Protein: 2.9g, Fat: 3.8g

Kale and Spinach Chips

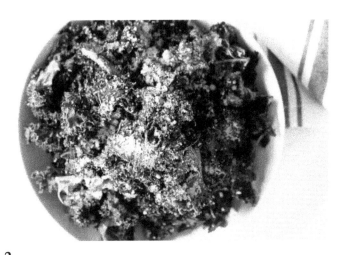

Serves: 2

Ingredients

- 2 cups spinach, torn in pieces and stem removed
- 2 cups kale, torn in pieces, stems removed
- 1 tablespoon of olive oil
- Sea salt, to taste
- 1/3 cup Parmesan cheese

Directions

1. Take a bowl and add spinach to it.
2. Take another bowl and add kale to it.
3. Now, season both of them with olive oil, and sea salt.
4. Add kale and spinach to the basket of the air fryer.
5. Select the air fry mode at 350 degrees F for 8 minutes.
6. Once done, take out the crispy chips and sprinkle Parmesan cheese on top.

Nutritional Information Per Serving: Calories 166| Fat 11.1g|
Sodium 355mg | Carbs 8.1g | Fiber1.7 g | Sugar 0.1g | Protein 8.2g

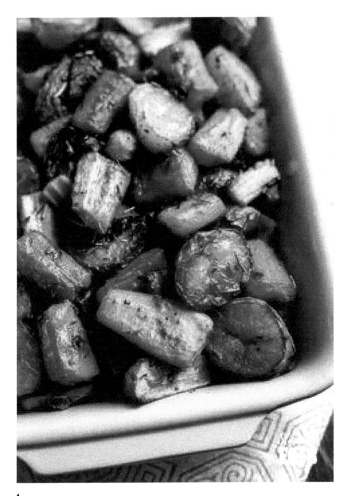

Serves: 4

Ingredients

- 2 cups of carrots, cubed

- 2 cups of potatoes, cubed

- 2 cups of shallots, cubed

- 2 cups zucchini, diced

- 2 cups yellow squash, cubed

- Salt and black pepper, to taste

- 1 tablespoon of Italian seasoning

- 2 tablespoons of ranch seasoning

- 4 tablespoons of olive oil

Directions

1. Take a large bowl and add all the veggies to it.

2. Season the veggies with salt, pepper, Italian seasoning, ranch seasoning, and olive oil

3. Toss all the ingredients well.

4. Now put it in the basket of the air fryer.

5. Set the unit to AIRFRY mode at 360 degrees F for 25 minutes.

6. Once it is cooked and done, serve, and enjoy.

Nutritional Information Per Serving: Calories 275| Fat 15.3g| Sodium129 mg | Carbs 33g | Fiber3.8 g | Sugar5 g | Protein 4.4g

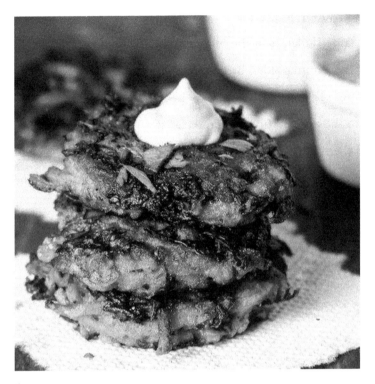

Serve 4:

Ingredients:

- 2 cups finely chopped potatoes
- 1 teaspoon extra-virgin olive oil or canola oil
- 1 clove garlic, minced
- 4 cups loosely packed coarsely chopped kale
- 1/8 cup almond milk
- 1/4 teaspoon sea salt
- 1/8 teaspoon ground black pepper
- Vegetable oil spray, as needed

Directions:

1. Add the potatoes to a large saucepan of boiling water. Cook until tender, about 30 minutes.

2. In a large skillet, heat the oil over medium-high heat. Add the garlic and sauté until golden brown. Add the kale and sauté for 2 to 3 minutes. Transfer to a large bowl.

3. Drain the cooked potatoes and transfer them to a medium bowl. Add the milk, salt, and pepper, and mash with a fork or potato masher. Transfer the potatoes to the large bowl and combine with the cooked kale.

4. Preheat the air fryer to 390°F for 5 minutes.

5. Roll the potato and kale mixture into 1-inch nuggets. Spritz the air fryer basket with vegetable oil. Place the nuggets in the air fryer and cook for 12 to 15 minutes, until golden brown, shaking at 6 minutes.

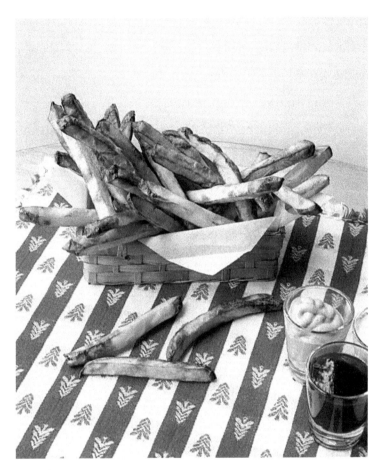

Serve 2 to 4:

Ingredients:

- 2 large russet potatoes, scrubbed
- 1/4 cup hot water
- 1 tablespoon Marmite or Vegemite
- 1 tablespoon apple cider vinegar

- Cut the potatoes into 1/4-inch slices, then cut the slices into 1/4-inch strips.

Directions:

1. Transfer the fries to a shallow baking pan or rimmed baking sheet.

2. Pour the water into a blender. Turn the blender on low and slowly drizzle in the Marmite. Add the vinegar, increase the blender's speed to high, and blend for just a few seconds. Pour the Marmite mixture over the fries. Toss the fries with tongs or use your hands to make sure the fries are coated with the marinade. Cover and set aside for about 15 minutes.

3. Preheat the air fryer to 360°F for 3 minutes. Drain the fries and transfer them to the air fryer. Cook at 360°F for 16 to 20 minutes, shaking halfway through the cooking time.

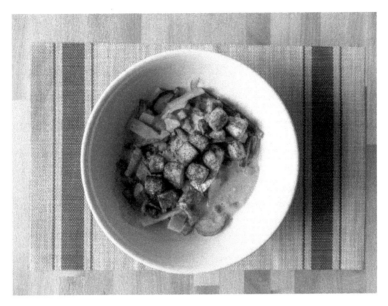

Serve 4:

Ingredients:

- 1 (14-ounce) package extra-firm tofu, frozen, thawed, drained, and pressed (see here)
- 1 teaspoon sesame oil
- 1/4 cup low-sodium soy sauce or tamari
- 2 tablespoons rice vinegar
- 2 teaspoons ground ginger, divided
- 2 teaspoons cornstarch or potato starch
- 1 teaspoon chickpea flour or brown rice flour

Directions:

1. Cut the block of tofu into 12 cubes and transfer them to an airtight container.

2. In a small bowl, whisk together the oil, soy sauce, vinegar, and 1 teaspoon of ginger. Pour the oil mixture over the cubed tofu, cover the container, and place in the refrigerator to marinate for at least 1 hour (ideally 8 hours).

3. Drain the marinated tofu and transfer it to a medium bowl. In a small bowl, combine the cornstarch, chickpea flour, and the remaining 1 teaspoon ginger. Sprinkle the cornstarch mixture over the drained tofu and gently toss with tongs, coating all the pieces of tofu.

4. Transfer the tofu to the air fryer. Cook at 350°F for 20 minutes. Shake at 10 minutes.

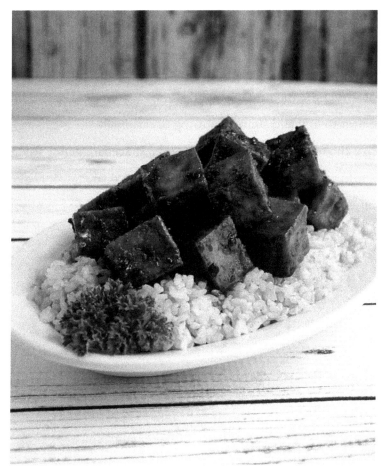

Serve 4:

Ingredients:

- Basic Air-Fried Tofu
- 1/4 cup low-sodium soy sauce
- 1/4 cup water
- 1/8 cup sugar

- 3 cloves garlic, minced
- 1/4 teaspoon ground ginger

Directions:

1. While the tofu is cooking in the air fryer, combine the soy sauce, water, sugar, garlic, and ginger in a saucepan over medium-high heat. Bring the mixture to a gentle boil, then immediately reduce the heat to low and simmer, stirring occasionally.

2. When the tofu is done, transfer it to the saucepan, gently folding the tofu into the sauce until all the cubes are coated. Cover and simmer on low for about 5 minutes (or until the tofu has absorbed the sauce).

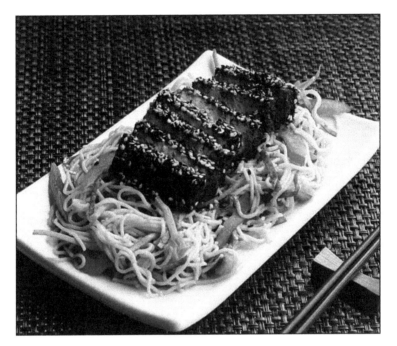

Serve 4:

Ingredients:

- 1 (14-ounce) package extra-firm tofu, frozen, thawed, drained, and pressed (see here)

- 1/4 cup tamari or soy sauce

- 1/8 cup rice vinegar

- 1/8 cup mirin (see note)

- 2 teaspoons sesame oil

- 2 teaspoons light or dark agave syrup or vegan honey

- 2 teaspoons minced garlic

- 1 teaspoon grated fresh ginger

- 1 to 2 spritzes canola oil
- 2 tablespoons black sesame seeds
- 2 tablespoons white sesame seeds
- 1 teaspoon potato starch

Directions:

1. Place the tofu in an airtight container that is about the size of the block of tofu so that the marinade completely covers it. In a small bowl, combine the tamari, vinegar, mirin, sesame oil, agave, garlic, and ginger. Pour the marinade over the tofu, cover the container, and refrigerate for 1 to 8 hours (the longer the better).

2. Remove the tofu from the container and cut it in half lengthwise. Then cut each half in half lengthwise to form 4 tofu steaks. Rub both sides of each piece in the marinade.

3. Spritz the air fryer basket with canola oil. Preheat the air fryer to 390°F for 3 minutes.

4. Sprinkle the black sesame seeds, white sesame seeds, and potato starch on a large plate. Combine well. Press a tofu steak into the seeds, flip over, and press the other side of the tofu into the seeds. Place the tofu in the air fryer basket and gently pat the seeds on top of the tofu into place. Add more seeds, if necessary, gently patting them into the tofu. Set the tofu slice aside on the plate.

5. Spritz the top of the tofu with additional canola oil. Cook at 390°F for 15 minutes. After about 7 minutes, gently use tongs to check that the tofu isn't sticking. (Do not flip the tofu!)

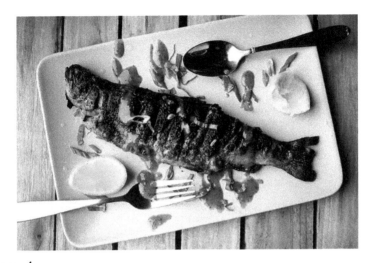

Serves: 4

Ingredients:

- 4 trout fillets

- 2 tablespoons olive oil

- ½ teaspoon salt

- 1 teaspoon black pepper

- 2 garlic cloves, sliced

- 1 lemon, sliced, plus additional wedges for serving

Directions:

1. . Preheat the air fryer to 380°F.

2. . Brush each fillet with olive oil on both sides and season with salt and pepper. Place the fillets in an even layer in the air fryer basket.

3. . Place the sliced garlic over the tops of the trout fillets, then top the garlic with lemon slices and cook for 12 to 15 minutes, or until it has reached an internal temperature of 145°F.

4. . Serve with fresh lemon wedges.

PER SERVING: Calories: 231; Total Fat: 12g; Saturated Fat: 2g;

Protein: 29g; Total Carbohydrates: 1g; Fiber: 0g; Sugar: 0g; Cholesterol:

84mg

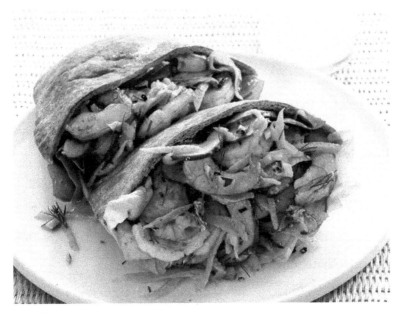

Serves: 2

Ingredients:

- 1 pound medium shrimp, peeled and deveined
- 2 tablespoons olive oil
- 1 teaspoon dried oregano
- ½ teaspoon dried thyme
- ½ teaspoon garlic powder
- ¼ teaspoon onion powder
- ½ teaspoon salt
- ¼ teaspoon black pepper
- 4 whole wheat pitas
- 4 ounces feta cheese, crumbled

- 1 cup shredded lettuce

- 1 tomato, diced

- ¼ cup black olives, sliced

- 1 lemon

Directions:

1. . Preheat the oven to 380°F.

2. . In a medium bowl, combine the shrimp with olive oil, oregano, thyme, garlic powder, onion powder, salt, and black pepper.

3. . Pour shrimp in a single layer in the air fryer basket and cook for 6 to 8 minutes, or until cooked through.

4. . Remove from the air fryer and divide into warmed pitas with feta, lettuce, tomato, olives, and a squeeze of lemon.

PER SERVING: Calories: 395; Total Fat: 16g; Saturated Fat: 6g; Protein: 26g; Total Carbohydrates: 40g; Fiber: 5g; Sugar: 3g; Cholesterol: 168mg

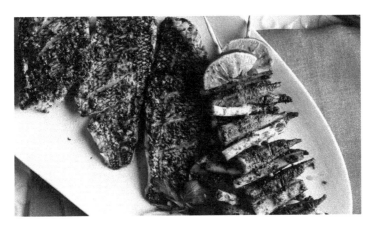

Serves: 4

Ingredients:

- 1 carrot, diced small

- 1 parsnip, diced small

- 1 rutabaga, diced small

- ¼ cup olive oil

- 2 teaspoons salt, divided

- 4 sea bass fillets

- ½ teaspoon onion powder

- 2 garlic cloves, minced

- 1 lemon, sliced, plus additional wedges for serving

Directions:

1. . Preheat the air fryer to 380°F.

2. . In a small bowl, toss the carrot, parsnip, and rutabaga with olive oil and 1 teaspoon salt.

3. . Lightly season the sea bass with the remaining 1 teaspoon of salt and the onion powder, then place it into the air fryer basket in a single layer.

4. . Spread the garlic over the top of each fillet, then cover with lemon slices.

5. . Pour the prepared vegetables into the basket around and on top of the fish. Roast for 15 minutes.

6. . Serve with additional lemon wedges if desired.

PER SERVING: Calories: 299; Total Fat: 16g; Saturated Fat: 3g; Protein: 25g; Total Carbohydrates: 13g; Fiber: 3g; Sugar: 5g; Cholesterol: 53mg

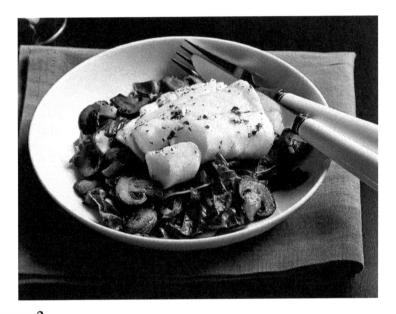

Serves: 2

Ingredients:

- 1 teaspoon salt
- ½ teaspoon dried oregano
- ½ teaspoon dried thyme
- ½ teaspoon garlic powder
- 4 cod fillets
- ½ white onion, thinly sliced
- 2 cups Swiss chard, washed, stemmed, and torn into pieces
- ¼ cup olive oil
- 1 lemon, quartered

Directions:

1. . Preheat the air fryer to 380°F.

2. . In a small bowl, whisk together the salt, oregano, thyme, and garlic powder.

3. . Tear off four pieces of aluminum foil, with each sheet being large enough to envelop one cod fillet and a quarter of the vegetables.

4. . Place a cod fillet in the middle of each sheet of foil, then sprinkle on all sides with the spice mixture.

5. . In each foil packet, place a quarter of the onion slices and ½ cup Swiss chard, then drizzle 1 tablespoon olive oil and squeeze ¼ lemon over the contents of each foil packet.

6. . Fold and seal the sides of the foil packets and then place them into the air fryer basket. Steam for 12 minutes.

7. . Remove from the basket, and carefully open each packet to avoid a steam burn.

PER SERVING: Calories: 252; Total Fat: 14g; Saturated Fat: 2g; Protein: 26g; Total Carbohydrates: 4g; Fiber: 1g; Sugar: 1g; Cholesterol: 61mg

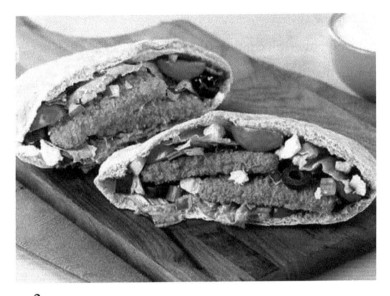

Serves: 2

Ingredients:

- 1 pound pollock, cut into 1-inch pieces
- ¼ cup olive oil
- 1 teaspoon salt
- ½ teaspoon dried oregano
- ½ teaspoon dried thyme
- ½ teaspoon garlic powder
- ¼ teaspoon cayenne
- 4 whole-wheat pitas
- 1 cup shredded lettuce
- 2 Roma tomatoes, diced
- Nonfat plain Greek yogurt

- Lemon, quartered

Directions:

1. . Preheat the air fryer to 380°F.

2. . In a medium bowl, combine the pollock with olive oil, salt, oregano, thyme, garlic powder, and cayenne.

3. . Put the pollock into the air fryer basket and cook for 15 minutes.

4. . Serve inside pitas with lettuce, tomato, and Greek yogurt with a lemon wedge on the side.

PER SERVING: Calories: 368; Total Fat: 16g; Saturated Fat: 2g; Protein: 21g; Total Carbohydrates: 38g; Fiber: 6g; Sugar: 2g; Cholesterol: 52mg

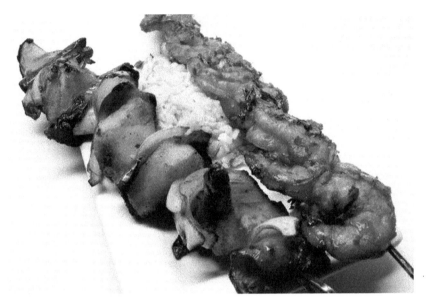

Serves: 12 skewered shrimp

Ingredients:

- 1½ tablespoons mirin
- 1½ teaspoons ginger juice
- 1½ tablespoons soy sauce
- 12 large shrimp (about 20 shrimps per pound), peeled and deveined
- 1 large egg
- ¾ cup panko bread crumbs
- Cooking spray

Directions:

1. Combine the mirin, ginger juice, and soy sauce in a large bowl. Stir to mix well.

2. Dunk the shrimp in the bowl of mirin mixture, then wrap the bowl in plastic and refrigerate for 1 hour to marinate.

3. Spritz the air fryer basket with cooking spray.

4. Run twelve 4-inch skewers through each shrimp.

5. Whisk the egg in the bowl of the marinade to combine well. Pour the bread crumbs on a plate.

6. Dredge the shrimp skewers in the egg mixture, then shake the excess off and roll over the bread crumbs to coat well.

7. Arrange the shrimp skewers in the basket and spritz with cooking spray.

8. Put the air fryer basket on the baking pan and slide into Rack Position 2, select Air Fry, set temperature to 400°F (205°C), and set time to 6 minutes.

9. Flip the shrimp skewers halfway through the cooking time.

10. When done, the shrimp will be opaque and firm.

11. Serve immediately.

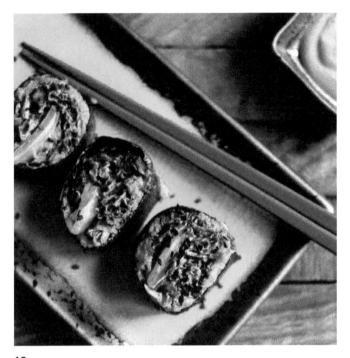

Serves: 12

Ingredients:

Kale Salad:

- 1½ cups chopped kale
- 1 tablespoon sesame seeds
- ¾ teaspoon soy sauce
- ¾ teaspoon toasted sesame oil
- ½ teaspoon rice vinegar
- ¼ teaspoon ginger
- ⅛ teaspoon garlic powder

Sushi Rolls:

- 3 sheets sushi nori
- 1 batch cauliflower rice
- ½ avocado, sliced
- Sriracha Mayonnaise:
- ¼ cup Sriracha sauce
- ¼ cup vegan mayonnaise

  Coating:
- ½ cup panko bread crumbs

Directions:

1. In a medium bowl, toss all the ingredients for the salad together until well coated and set aside.
2. Place a sheet of nori on a clean work surface and spread the cauliflower rice in an even layer on the nori. Scoop 2 to 3 tablespoon of kale salad on the rice and spread over. Place 1 or 2 avocado slices on top. Roll up the sushi, pressing gently to get a nice, tight roll. Repeat to make the remaining 2 rolls.
3. In a bowl, stir together the Sriracha sauce and mayonnaise until smooth. Add bread crumbs to a separate bowl.
4. Dredge the sushi rolls in Sriracha Mayonnaise, then roll in bread crumbs till well coated.
5. Place the coated sushi rolls in the air fryer basket.
6. Put the air fryer basket on the baking pan and slide into Rack Position 2, select Air Fry, set temperature to 390°F (199°C), and set time to 10 minutes.
7. Flip the sushi rolls halfway through the cooking time.

8. When cooking is complete, the sushi rolls will be golden brown and crispy...

9. Transfer to a platter and rest for 5 minutes before slicing each roll into 8 pieces. Serve warm.

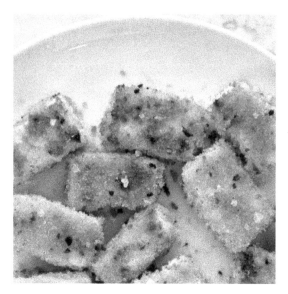

Serves: 20 nuggets

Ingredients:

- 1 cup all-purpose flour, plus more for dusting
- 1 teaspoon baking powder
- ½ teaspoon butter, at room temperature, plus more for brushing
- ¼ teaspoon salt
- ¼ cup water
- ⅛ teaspoon onion powder
- ¼ teaspoon garlic powder
- ⅛ teaspoon seasoning salt
- Cooking spray

Directions:

1. Line the air fryer basket with parchment paper.

2. Mix the flour, baking powder, butter, and salt in a large bowl. Stir to mix well. Gradually whisk in the water until a sanity dough forms.

3. Put the dough on a lightly floured work surface, then roll it out into a ½-inch thick rectangle with a rolling pin.

4. Cut the dough into about twenty 1- or 2-inch squares, then arrange the squares in a single layer in the basket. Spritz with cooking spray.

5. Combine onion powder, garlic powder, and seasoning salt in a small bowl. Stir to mix well, then sprinkle the squares with the powder mixture.

6. Put the air fryer basket on the baking pan and slide into Rack Position 2, select Air Fry, set temperature to 370°F (188°C), and set time to 4 minutes.

7. Flip the squares halfway through the cooking time.

8. When cooked, the dough squares should be golden brown.

9. Remove the golden nuggets from the oven and brush with more butter immediately. Serve warm.

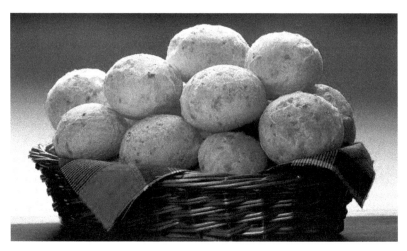

Serves: 12 balls

Ingredients:

- 2 tablespoons butter, plus more for greasing
- ½ cup milk
- 1½ cups tapioca flour
- ½ teaspoon salt
- 1 large egg
- ⅔ cup finely grated aged Asiago cheese

Directions:

1. Put the butter in a saucepan and pour in the milk, heat over medium heat until the liquid boils. Keep stirring.

2. Turn off the heat and mix in the tapioca flour and salt to form a soft dough. Transfer the dough to a large bowl, then wrap the bowl in plastic and let sit for 15 minutes.

3. Break the egg in the bowl of dough and whisk with a hand mixer for 2 minutes or until a sanity dough forms. Fold the cheese in the dough. Cover the bowl in plastic again and let sit for 10 more minutes.

4. Grease the baking pan with butter.

5. Scoop 2 tablespoons of the dough into the baking pan. Repeat with the remaining dough to make dough 12 balls. Keep a little distance between every two balls.

6. Slide the baking pan into Rack Position 1, select Convection Bake set the temperature to 375°F (190°C), and set time to 12 minutes.

7. Flip the balls halfway through the cooking time.

8. When cooking is complete, the balls should be golden brown and fluffy.

9. Remove the balls from the oven and allow to cool for 5 minutes before serving.

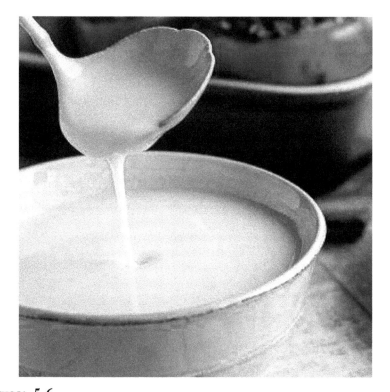

Serves: 5-6

Ingredients:

- 5 ounces Cheddar cheese, sliced
- 1/5 tsp sodium citrate
- 1/3 cup water

Directions:

1. Set your cooking device to 167 degrees F.
2. Carefully place the ingredients into the vacuum bag, seal the bag and cook in the preheated water bath for 20 minutes.

3. When the time is up, pour the sauce into a bowl and blend with an immersion blender until even.

Nutrition per serving: Calories: 80, Protein: 3 g, Fats: 5 g, Carbs: 4 g

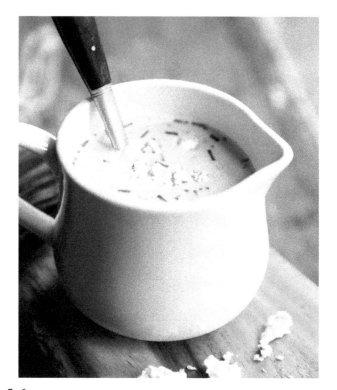

Serves: 5-6

Ingredients:

- 5 ounces blue cheese, crumbled
- 1/5 tsp sodium citrate
- 1/3 cup water

Directions:

1. Set your cooking device to 167 degrees F.
2. Carefully place the ingredients into the vacuum bag, seal the bag and cook in the preheated water bath for 20 minutes.

3. When the time is up, pour the sauce into a bowl and blend with an immersion blender until even.

Nutrition per serving: Calories: 73, Protein: 2 g, Fats: 6 g, Carbs: 2 g

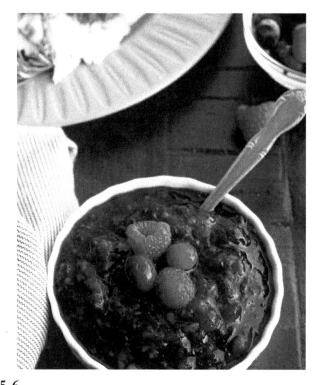

Serves: 5-6

Ingredients:

- 1 cup fresh cranberries
- Zest of 1/2 orange
- 7 tbsp white sugar

Directions:

1. Set your cooking device to 194 degrees F.
2. Carefully place the ingredients into the vacuum bag, seal the bag and cook in the preheated water bath for 2 hours.

3. When the time is up, pour the sauce into a sauceboat and serve with lamb or beef.

Nutrition per serving: Calories: 54, Protein: 0.2 g, Fats: 0.4 g, Carbs: 14 g

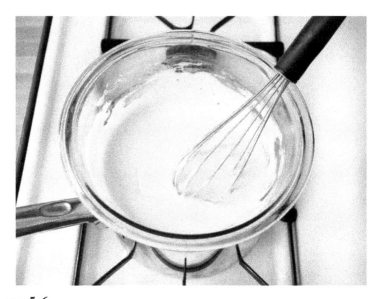

Serves: 5-6

Ingredients:

- 1/5 cup white wine vinegar
- 2 shallots, finely chopped
- 1/2 cup butter
- 4 egg yolks
- 1/5 cup still water
- 1 tbsp lemon juice A pinch of salt

Directions:

1. Put the finely chopped shallots into a small saucepan, add the white wine vinegar and simmer until the liquid is reduced by half.

2. Set your cooking device to 185 degrees F.

3. Carefully pour the cooked shallots with the vinegar into the vacuum bag, add all other ingredients, seal the bag and cook in the preheated water bath for 30 minutes.
4. When the time is up, pour the sauce into a bowl, blend with an immersion blender and serve.

Nutrition per serving: Calories: 161, Protein: 2 g, Fats: 15 g, Carbs: 4.5 g

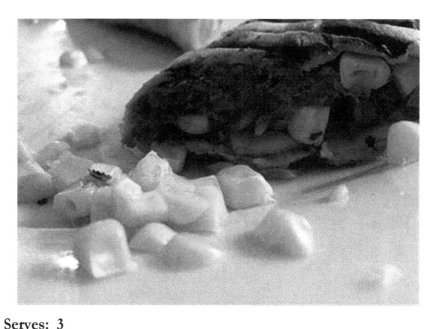

Serves: 3

Ingredients

- 1½ kg Pork neck without bones

- 2½ tsp Five-spice powder

- ¼ cup hoisin sauce

- 3 tbsp. soy sauce

- 3 tbsp. honey

- 2 tbsp. Rice wine (Shaoxing rice wine)

- 2 tbsp. Ginger, fresher, grated

- 2 tbsp. Garlic, pressed

- 1 Lemon, peel thereof

Directions

1. You need Air Fryer cooker, a vacuum device, and a vacuum bag. I suppose you can use a very dense freezer bag, but I wouldn't trust the density.

2. If you have got the pork neck with bone, you either have to remove it or put two bags on top of each other for Air Fryer cooking so that the bone does not cut a hole in the bag and water gets into it.

3. Either leave the pork neck whole or cut it into rough cubes. The advantage of the previous cutting is that the length of the meat fibers is already determined.

4. Mix the remaining ingredients for the marinade sauce.

5. Now cut a bag into a sufficiently large size for Air Fryer cooking and be generous. Already weld a seam with the vacuum sealer and put the meat in the opening of the bag.

6. Pour in the sauce and vacuum the bag - being careful not to remove the sauce.

7. Put enough water in the Air Fryer cooker at 70 ° C. When the temperature is reached, put the bag in so that it is completely submerged. Tip: I always add hot water to save time. Leave the meat in a water bath for 20 - 24 hours.

8. In the meantime, be sure to check whether there is still enough liquid and, above all, whether the bag is floating off the meat due to the development of steam. If so, you have to complain and press under the surface. Cutlery, tongs, etc. can be used for this - just nothing, please, that keeps the water away from the meat, such as plates and the like.

9. Optional: For a light crust, preheat the oven to maximum temperature and grill or top heat.

10. After cooking, remove the bag, cut a small corner, and pour the leaked liquid into a saucepan. Remove the meat from the bag. Now it is theoretically finished and can be picked up.

11. Or for a light crust, pat the meat dry on the outside. Place in a large ovenproof dish and grill in the oven until a light crust has formed. Then shred the meat in a large bowl. That should be very easy. Now add the zest of the lemon.

12. Try the meat: if it is too dry, add some of the liquid. Otherwise, gently boil down the leaked liquid on the stove.

13. To do this, you have to use a heat-resistant silicone spatula to stir constantly and move the sauce at the bottom of the pot, because the liquid contains honey and hoisin sauce - both tend to burn.

14. When the desired consistency is achieved, the sauce can be added to the meat and mixed in or served separately. I usually mix them in. The mixture can also be loosened up well with a little water.

15. This "Pulled Pork" in the Asian style is quite sweet and can now be eaten in any way: on burger rolls, in wraps, tacos, etc.

16. The meat is particularly good with something crisp, as well as with a little acid, such as something inlaid. For example, I take a few cucumber slices that have been briefly soaked in a vinegar-water-sugar-salt mixture of red onions that have been sliced with a pinch of salt and sugar, and light vinegar with a fork, or classic coleslaw. I also find corn and spring onions very nice.

17. Freezing works easily right after Air Fryer cooking. Quickly cool down, re-vacuum, and freeze while still in the bag in the ice bath.

18. Use within about 4 weeks.

19. To do this, defrost the meat gently in the refrigerator over 2 days, then place it under the grill or fry it all around in the pan. This only works if the meat is cold and therefore firmer than straight from the Air Fryer cooker. Then pick them up and, if necessary, bring them back to full temperature in the microwave or a saucepan.

20. The amount is for 4 people - from 1.5 kg after Air Fryer cooking approx. 1.1 kg - is generously calculated and varies depending on the purpose.

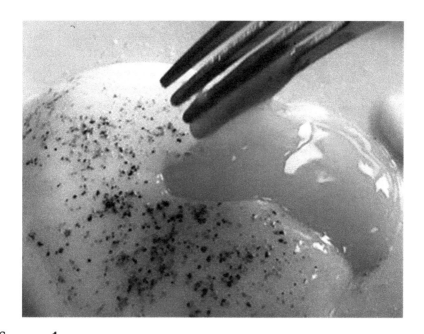

Serves: 1

Ingredients

- 1 Egg, size L
- 1 pinch salt and pepper

Directions

1. I have set the Air Fryer stick to 62 ° C. Then place the egg or eggs in a water bath for 45 minutes.

2. At the temperature I set, the egg yolk is still very fluid - which is why it can also be used as a topping for pasta or other dishes. The egg yolk is firmer at approx. 68 ° C and does not run all over the plate.

3. After cooking, quench the egg under cold water, whip it with a knife, and put it on the plate. Refine with salt, pepper, and other spices as you like.

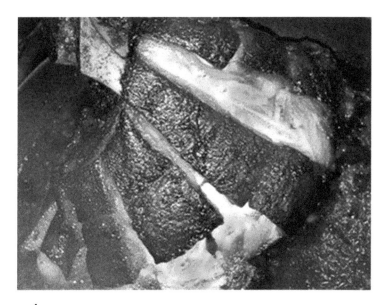

Serves: 1

Ingredients

- 1 Pork knuckle or knuckle of pork
- Spice at will

Directions

1. The fresh, uncured pork knuckle, also known elsewhere as the knuckle of pork or in Austria as stilts, is washed, dried, and put in a vacuum bag.

2. This is followed by spices at will. I like to use a grill spice mix of bell peppers (spicy and sweet), pepper, garlic, salt, and a little sugar. Then the air is extracted as far as possible and the bag is sealed airtight. I use a vacuum device for this (it should also be possible to remove

the air in another way and seal the bag securely. I have no experience with that.)

3. Now the bag goes into a water bath for 28 hours at 70 degrees Celsius.

4. After the bath, the shank is removed from the pouch and the skin of the shank is cut into a diamond shape. The knuckle is placed in a saucepan and poured with the liquid from the bag.

5. Now the rind is crispy fried in the oven at 160 degrees Celsius in about 45 minutes and a butter-tender but crispy knuckle is finished.

Index

A

B

C

D

E

G

H

K

L

M

P

S

T

U

Cooking Conversion Chart

TEMPERATURE		WEIGHT	
FAHRENHEIT	**CELSIUS**	**IMPERIAL**	**METRIC**
100 °F	37 °C	1/2 oz	15 g
150 °F	65 °C	1 oz	29 g
200 °F	93 °C	2 oz	57 g
250 °F	121 °C	3 oz	85 g
300 °F	150 °C	4 oz	113 g
325 °F	160 °C	5 oz	141 g
350 °F	180 °C	6 oz	170 g
375 °F	190 °C	8 oz	227 g
400 °F	200 °C	10 oz	283 g
425 °F	220 °C	12 oz	340 g
450 °F	230 °C	13 oz	369 g
500 °F	260 °C	14 oz	397 g
525 °F	270 °C	15 oz	425 g
550 °F	288 °C	1 lb	453 g

MEASUREMENT			
CUP	ONCES	MILLILITERS	TABLESPOON
1/16 cup	1/2 oz	15 ml	1
1/8 cup	1 oz	30 ml	3
1/4 cup	2 oz	59 ml	4
1/3 cup	2.5 oz	79 ml	5.5
3/8 cup	3 oz	90 ml	6
1/2 cup	4 oz	118 ml	8
2/3 cup	5 oz	158 ml	11
3/4 cup	6 oz	177 ml	12
1 cup	8 oz	240 ml	16
2 cup	16 oz	480 ml	32
4 cup	32 oz	960 ml	64
5 cup	40 oz	1180 ml	80
6 cup	48 oz	1420 ml	96
8 cup	64 oz	1895 ml	128

CPSIA information can be obtained
at www.ICGtesting.com
Printed in the USA
LVHW050601280621
691310LV00007B/211